Title

HEALTH IS WEALTH

Subtitle

Make a Delectable Investment in You!

Table of Content

Title

HEALTH IS WEALTH

Subtitle

Make a Delectable Investment in You!

Table of Content

How can health be made more valuable?
Think This out this Basic Self-Care Advice:

CHAPTER 1

WHOLENESS IS WEALTH

"Health is Wealth," According to the proverb, riches is a condition of health free from disease or disorders, both bodily and mental. The saying "The Greatest Wealth is Health" by the great Classical Rome poet Virgil (Publius Vergilius Maro) indicates that the adage is old. Virgil has had poor health throughout his life, and it's conceivable that this fact motivated him to share this aphorism as a piece of wisdom with future generations. Similarly, a Spanish proverb says that a guy who is too busy to care for his health is like a mechanic who is too busy to care for his tools.

Why don't we take care of ourselves?

A while back, I was preparing a meal of black bean and quinoa dip for a gathering of friends and family while I was in the kitchen. I abruptly heard someone behind me ask, "What is that? I won't eat that, even if it's something healthy.

There was truth in what was stated, even though it was perhaps expressed partially in jest, just as there is in similar remarks that frequently go something like this: "My doctor says I have to start eating healthily since my numbers (i.e., cholesterol, blood pressure) are awful." Even in the doctor's waiting room, where medical professionals have spent a large portion of their careers learning about the benefits of a good diet, the remarks about healthy eating often sound like parents telling their young children it's time to go to bed.

But it's just not related to what we consume. A recent article from The Wall Street Journal examined the detrimental consequences that smartphones may have on our intelligence. Regarding our health and well-being, there is an ever-growing body of bad news concerning devices and usage habits. Many people would admit that, although enjoying the convenience and experience, having a smartphone with them all the time isn't exactly doing their physical and mental health any favors.

If we are being honest, these are only two of many instances where people (consciously or unconsciously) disregard their short- and long-term health in favor of instant gratification, convenience, and experience. Although we, as a culture, may act as though mental and physical health is of the utmost importance, our actions and routines consistently reflect the opposite. So why do we sacrifice our health and happiness for other rewards?

It can be tricky, just like most questions involving human behavior. To begin with, we should be aware that everyone defines "health" and "well-being" according to their standards and beliefs. A person's idea of health may differ from another person's definition of inactivity depending on how you were taught and who your current role models are. Lack of knowledge about healthy habits can also be a barrier, though this is less of an issue now that so much information is available.

Beyond varying standards and a lack of information, there are a few fundamental causes for why people's practices blatantly go against what they know to be healthy. First, leading a healthy lifestyle necessitates discipline; that is, to be completely honest and unappealing to some people. This discipline includes both strenuous activity and periodic abstinence. They believe it will just increase the stress and difficulties they already experience, which is one of the reasons it is unattractive (even if evidence suggests that in the long term, it might do the opposite). Going for a jog and skipping dessert may seem like the last things you want to do after a hard day at work and feeling mentally and physically drained.

The second barrier is connected to this. Although feeling healthy can be enjoyable, it rarely compares to the hedonistic thrill of a delicious ice cream cone or a sensational or absurd online feed. A collective focus that gradually develops within the person to satisfy urges and yearnings, but not necessarily because it evokes a complete thrill or an absolute sense of relief, is what good health practices entail. They are rarely like roller coasters or repeated Facebook messages. I satisfy a yearning (in addition to numerous FDA criteria) and my desire for calories when I eat my head-sized salad at dinner or my bowl of Grape Nuts before I go to bed. However, it will never be as commonplace as pizza and ice cream, even though I have no desire (indeed, yearning) to follow this routine.

If we dig deeper, one of the fundamental reasons we reject our health and well-being is that we have no faith that the process will genuinely take us somewhere happier and more fulfilling. One time, a coworker insisted on starting each day with a Coke (and probably ending with one, too). She was confident that Coke would give her a focused, dependable source of goodness no matter how demanding the day was. McDonald's is aware of this, which is why their cups and packaging frequently use the words "joy," "pleasure," and "peace." The issue with her Coke (and other such meals) contributed to her elevated anxiety and worsening health. She understood it because she works in health care.

Despite this, all the information could have been more helpful because eliminating the one surefire way to feel happy was highly uncomfortable. Not only did the pressures loom huge, but it also seemed like a pipe dream to assume that better thinking, more mental calm, and a healthier physique only result in more happiness and contentment. And this is how it is for most people, mainly if you have never actually known somebody who has had this experience. When we want to feel well immediately, mysterious improvements in health that take time appear like quite a risky undertaking. Our health is no different; it requires a leap of faith to achieve anything worthwhile. There are many opportunities to feel good and be healthy, but we must first decide what is most crucial in our lives. Quinoa will only be one of the things left over if we keep rejecting our health and well-being in favor of other rewards.

CHAPTER 2

Health Benefits

The advantages of good health include the following:

Overall well-being
Increasing the potential for extended life decreased the likelihood of depression.
I have more robust bones and muscles.
I am getting to or keeping a healthy weight.

What is more than my general welfare, we must ask ourselves? Exercise in the morning, consume healthy meals, adopt a healthy lifestyle, and resist peer pressure.

When personal self-care is neglected due to the busyness of life, it can hurt a person's overall health and wellness. People today balance their jobs, home, traffic, and social commitments, which hurts their health and reminds them that no aspect of self-care should be disregarded.

As individuals, we must learn what is best for us and consciously make small changes that align us to be our best, "healthiest" selves. Health is an investment.

A run over an 'unnecessary' meeting, wholesome food over less-healthy options, and a conscious corporation over a mindless profit-hungry one are all things we should prioritize over our health.

We are entirely answerable for the condition of our bodies and our health. Focusing on self-care practices will enhance our general quality of life and health since repetition creates habits.

Let's look at some basic routines that can help you maintain a healthy balance between your physical, mental, and emotional well-being. They may even make it more enjoyable.

Be aware of your self-worth: A person's confidence and self-esteem will increase once they grasp how crucial it is to elicit pleasant emotions.

Keep a healthy work-life balance: Stress and tiredness can result from an overworked lifestyle and may result in a less fulfilling, unorganized, and emotionally draining life. Work more wisely.

Management of stress: Long-term stress and anxiety negatively impact mental and physical health. Make it a practice to unwind.

Live life with greater zeal: Setting aside time each day to take care of oneself (by having a quick shower, reading, drawing, learning a new activity, etc.) not only recharges but also provides new inspiration and justification for rising early.

Physical well-being: Self-care practices that promote physical well-being include regular exercise, a good diet, and enough sleep.

Steps to Make Health Your Wealth

For the vast majority, wealth means owning a lot of cash, a sizable plot of land, expensive jewelry, a car, a farm, a flat, a house, or any other type of property that might be sold for a profit. Although the term "wealth" is perfectly appropriate in its traditional sense and according to the dictionary definition, this restricts its range and perspective. However, if we expand our perspective and go beyond our narrow view of "Wealth," we will realize and experience that wealth is not just what is being said about it. Let's look at our own lives to understand this better.

Although "Knowledge" and "Experience," like currency, cannot be touched or felt, they are nonetheless a form of wealth that we accumulate in school, college, or the workplace. In this case, it is wealth because it has a valid, regarded, and admired value in various social settings. Additionally, by applying "Unconventional Wealth," you can increase your wealth. There are several different types of unconventional.

Health is the essence of wealth, roughly on par with "Spiritual Health," and it is the source of all other forms of wealth and highlights that "Wealth" is dependent on and connected to "Health" in more ways than one. For instance, if you are physically and mentally ill, you will not be able to work effectively or at all. And you won't be able to accumulate the necessary level of riches if you can't work in the intended way. Health cannot be inversely related to income because being healthy requires very little money unless you pay to receive training to stay in shape. Having stated that it is not advisable to be "Wealthy" to be "Healthy," you should avoid becoming so focused on your health that it hinders your ability to produce riches. Those who genuinely view health as wealth and not merely a trend understand its importance and how much wealth it is. Those who have yet to grasp this should do so.

CHAPTER 3

What is the resource you value the most?

Why health is more important than riches, according to The Bottom Line Isn't What You Think It Is.....
Many people instantly associate the term **"valuable"** with money or wealth when they hear it. A recent Forbes article claims that while most successful people name time their most valuable asset, finances get a solid, honorable mention. If it's not top of mind, it's close.

But when it comes to worth, I'd like to recommend moving health up to the top rank for the following reasons:

You must have good health to obtain all other precious resources. You can only build wealth if you are in good health. I'm not simply referring to money, either. It is more difficult to accumulate a wealth of life experiences and take care of your spiritual and emotional health when dealing with a debilitating physical condition or a persistent lack of access to the resources for healthy living. The more time we spend on surviving, the less time we have to focus on thriving. When our energy is consistently consumed to achieve or maintain a basic level of health, there is little left to devote to achieving anything else.

The prerequisite for enjoying any other priceless treasure is good health. In truth, health is considered equal to material assets. According to a study, the lack of health will prevent the individual, family, and community from falling behind on the wealth scale. Your state of health allows you to take advantage of all that life offers and build memories that are frequently more treasured than material possessions. One example of people's increased importance on creating memories over merely acquiring a luxury item is the surge in the popularity of experiencing vacations.

It comprehends how everything else flows from health; it is necessary to understand health holistically. Physical well-being is only one aspect of your overall health; the other three are also important. What you do for this cohesive whole you refer to as Your experience of riches is directly influenced by you. Even though they may be wealthy, a "toxic" person who disrespects their own body and mistreats others will never be able to enjoy thankfulness and joy since their ability to do so will be impaired. Contrast this with someone who treats others with compassion and respects their body, mind, and spirit. This person will view wealth as a blessing and most likely share it, continuing the cycle of good health and goodwill.

Most things can be purchased with money, but health cannot. Treatments may be purchased, but the quality of life—the capacity to feel joy and spread it to others—cannot be purchased. The best approach to being wealthy is taking care of your physical, mental, and spiritual well-being just as you would your finances or source of income.

It turns out that the way to a life of prosperity is the same as the path to a life of holistic health:

Eat properly.

Keep a practical perspective on life.

Nourish your mind and soul.

Be grateful for whatever you have.

Smile frequently.

Be kind.

If you do, you could be surprised by how wealthy you are.

CHAPTER 4

8 Reasons Why Your Health Is Your Most Valuable Asset

The Additional Advantages of Maintaining a Healthy Lifestyle (from a financial perspective)

1. MEDICAL CHARGES CAN BE HIGH.

Medical expenses are lower for healthy persons. People who are ill spend their hard-earned money on medical expenses rather than enjoyable activities. Are all illnesses and injuries curable? Of course not, but the stock market is also not collapsing. The impact of unanticipated circumstances will only throw everything off course if you position yourself for success.

2. PRODUCTIVE WORKERS ARE HEALTHY WORKERS.

We can work more effectively when we are healthy. According to studies, good health workers can work harder and earn more money. Being kind to yourself will make you kind to everyone around you.

3. YOU GAIN CONFIDENCE WHEN YOU FEEL GREAT.

A high degree of wellness is accompanied by a confident and determined attitude to help you achieve your goals.

4. THE COST OF HEALTH INSURANCE IS INCREASING.

In the US, the cost of health insurance is already exorbitantly expensive. Constantly seeing a doctor will drive up those expenditures and detract from your ability to reach your financial objectives.

5. WORKOUTS ARE FREE.

Any wise businessman will tell you that you have profited if you provide nothing but receive a lot in return. Running, doing yoga in your living room, or dancing are all forms of exercise that are entirely free yet significantly improve your physical and mental health, as well as your financial situation. Additionally, there are a ton of free online tools and fitness instructors that can be viewed on YouTube. Take up a challenge right now!

6. PRODUCTIVENESS LASTS LONGER IN THE HEALTHY.

Healthy energy levels are frequently required because earning money requires energy. You can continue making money later in life if you practice good, healthful habits.

7. GOOD HEALTH INCREASES BRAIN POWER.

Consuming foods substantial in zinc, omega fatty acids, and other essential nutrients help your brain function at its best.

8. A HEALTH INVESTMENT IS.

Spending money on sneakers, smoothies, supplements, and other items is possible.

However, this is a financial commitment that may ultimately benefit you.

CHAPTER 5

Health is called wealth, but why?

Because of the many benefits of being healthy, some of which may not have yet been fully appreciated—health is wealth. The advantages obtained directly attest to this fact's veracity and confirm its accuracy.

The foundation of all other wealth is health. There are several connections between health and money. But one aspect stands out above the rest: health encourages prosperity. As a result of being more energetic, intelligent, and practical, a healthy person will be able to work harder and make more money, which may be used to enhance their efforts to accumulate wealth.

Health is a Good Investment with Long-Term Benefits: Health is a good investment with long-term benefits, and it is clear from the fact that - People with poor health frequently pass away at a young age. They have been neglecting their health in favor of accumulating cash. Their "Career Life" was victorious, but since they are no longer with us, it was a waste. In addition, many people need to survive longer to receive the pension and other benefits they worked for; At the same time, death is unavoidable and unexpected; leading a healthy lifestyle reduces your risk of passing away young from a sickness. In contrast, a healthy individual is more likely to live longer and benefit from their labor both in the short and long term. A healthy lifestyle will protect them from most diseases, and they may even leave behind cash that will be advantageous to their successors and survivors.

Healthy population Supports a Healthy Economy: A country's well-developed economy is directly supported by its healthy population.

It is simple to comprehend that if an organization's personnel are ill or unwell, its revenues will decline or stay the same and will impact the organization and the money made from these. Only when a nation's underlying infrastructure is sound can its economy grow. The outcome will be better the better each component of the structure is. The World Health Organization's most recent study serves as an illustration of this point. The study estimates that 47% of the workforce is overweight in urbanized industrial settings. Around 10% of individuals surveyed have diabetes, while about 27% have hypertension. The study found that people in the workforce have a higher risk of contracting chronic illnesses like obesity, heart disease, stroke, and cancer. To envision the potential of such an industrial setup, one can use the expertise of an expert.

Better Living through Health: Being in good health naturally increases our body's capability and ability to take advantage of possibilities to earn more money and live better. It makes one a better person, both intellectually and physically; personal happiness and healthy living with good values like diligence, generosity, kindness, discipline, and other desirable traits are encouraged by a healthy mentality. However, an unhealthy lifestyle contributes to a miserable existence. Even though a wealthy person may have all the comforts of life, that doesn't guarantee that he is leading a happy life. Only by realizing that "Health is a means to Better Living," in terms of infrastructure and mentality, can one live a better life.

Healthy mind Stays in a Healthy Body: It is undeniably true that leading a healthy lifestyle also contributes to mental abilities such as creativity, humor, presence of mind, humility, presentation, and communication. Our brain is stimulated and energized by a healthy, active body, which is made possible by a physical regimen, a balanced diet, meditation, and prayer. It improves brain function across the board, allowing one to excel and motivate others to follow in their footsteps.

Exercise is the Best Medicine, but it hasn't always been said that way. Prevention is always better than cure. The saying is still true today: regular exercise significantly reduces the risk of contracting any sickness. Physical, mental, and spiritual exercise boosts our immune systems and builds us up. Infections, allergies, stress, and other health issues will be less likely to harm us.
Furthermore, it supports the adage **"Prevention is Better than Cure."** If we had adhered to the fundamental rule, we could have avoided spending money and time on trips and purchasing medication. Most of us don't care for our health; we usually only focus on the more significant issue when we are harmed. The treatment has a cost and may adversely affect a

person's health. For instance, financial strain can result in physical symptoms of stress like migraines, insomnia, and anxiety due to high costs or unpaid medical bills. A person is more prone to experience financial trouble if they already need money. Long-lasting effects like lousy credit history, bankruptcy, and reduced income can make things even more difficult. Prevention strategies like regular exercise, sound sleep, a healthy diet, regular checkups, etc., are preferable to the results of breaking this straightforward rule of life.

Good health is a **"Beneficial Money Saving Scheme"** because the money that would have been spent on medical expenses and other related costs to treat ailments has been saved and used to make additional savings. Numerous cases exist where people become insolvent and destitute due to medical treatment. They could have avoided spending money if they had listened and acted upon the excellent advice.

Prevention of Anti-Social Behavior and Bad Habits: People who lead healthy lifestyles tend to have lessened or no alcoholism, smoking, drug usage, and other criminal tendencies. When one is "Money Minded," undesirable emotions such as greed, envy, anger, and desire for vengeance often worsen. Such people only care about getting what they want, no matter the cost. Their brains are tainted and centered on accumulating vast wealth; this inclination encourages other bad habits that even the untainted mind is susceptible to; however, the results are always harmful, even for people who are not closely related to the individual who committed the act. Because of their intellectual mind, a healthy person is aware of the consequences and, as a result, will not only refrain from them but actively work to prevent them for the benefit of society. People who have survived such events are already seasoned and unwilling to repeat the same mistakes.

Increases Life Fulfillment: Health is one factor that includes all the beneficial aspects that can increase life satisfaction. People with sound minds know how to manage their financial and physical well-being. It can be seen in their actions and attitudes. Healthy people are more likely to lead better lives than those who aren't. Only when we have the time and energy can we truly appreciate everything life offers. A sense of well-being fosters an atmosphere in which one can concentrate on all aspects of his life without worry or tension. Even a tiny green leaf might bring joy to someone in good health.

A healthier society is created by having healthy individuals. Balanced people follow the laws, foster peace, collaborate, are responsible, participate in volunteer work, and engage in productive activities and other worthwhile activities that improve society and establish or restore social decorum. The only time a person will consider others in society is when they are content with their own life. Similar feelings are indirectly and explicitly encouraged by these people's actions and conduct among all age groups.

CHAPTER 6

Why don't we abide by the Wise Counsel?

Health is something we take for granted and sometimes don't even think about, like other good laws of life that are meant to be followed. Some people still have time to take action, while others cannot. Whatever the circumstance or attitude, human nature's propensity to gravitate toward ease and comfort breeds terrible traits.

Career-Driven Life: Whether intentionally or unintentionally, we choose a career when weighing it against our health. Our careers have been emphasized as the one important goal we must accomplish throughout our lives. However, we neglect to emphasize the enormous potential that good health has for our daily lives and careers. Health is sometimes wholly disregarded when the message of the career is louder. Thus begins a career life where people must sit for extended periods, labor like ants, and are also taken advantage of. Wein lives under work alone; we cannot meet our needs for exercise, nutrition, entertainment, and other daily chores. When we even go the extra mile and work non-stop for days to make ends meet. Working hard is not terrible, but it is not appropriate to do so at the expense of our health and lives. When will we have time to enjoy achievement if we keep working and don't strike a balance between work and health? People who lead this lifestyle tend to be overweight, hypertensive, and frail.

Lack of Time: This is the most typical justification for not having enough time to devote to one's health and is valid for many of us; we are so engrossed in the work that we hurry through and limit daily tasks like laundry, having a healthy meal, or missing breakfast. Additionally, we frequently engage in demeaning activities such as inappropriate late-night gatherings, parties, and fast food. Health is not even on the list because of our busy schedules. We are so preoccupied with this that we don't even have time to think about or make time for it in our schedules. As a result, we completely abandoned the plan. Time will always be available; we need good management and dedication.

Disease-Free = Healthy: A significant portion of the population believes that if they are disease-free, they are healthy and don't need to worry about anything. Being disease-free alone is nice, but keeping the body that way will eventually take work. Everything around us has life; therefore, until and unless we take the necessary actions, this state of being disease-free will likewise not last very long. Not to mention that just because you don't think you have a sickness doesn't mean you do. Attend routine checkups to avoid having the wrong impression.

Youth Mentality: The typical attitude among young people is, "I'm youthful; I don't need any exercise." They also find exercise and similar activities tedious, dull, and time-consuming. Teenagers and their peers typically have good health since they lead structured lives that include physical activity. It is untrue, though, that you don't need to exercise if you're young. Regular physical and mental exercise improves and strengthens a person. A routine established at this period develops a habit one may maintain throughout life.

Urbanization and technology-fueled urbanization have made us lazy. We have servants who do our daily tasks, we commute in cars because it saves us time, we eat fast food because we don't want to cook, and we sit in front of our computers or televisions playing video games or watching reality shows. These things have contributed to our complacency and inactive lifestyle over time. We don't like to work hard because it seems archaic in our ready-made society, especially since we have the technology to carry out our jobs.

Shortcuts: A new generation of health goods that promise to make you healthy while you sit in your homes have been saturating the market. We have body toning devices, sauna belts, figure enhancers, herbal teas, and other things. All of them not only encourage idleness but also suggest that quick fixes to good health are possible. But there is no shortcut to hard work; the only shortcut is hard labor. These items are supplemental in nature and untrustworthy. There are no substitutes for traditional forms of exercise.

Servants of our Habits: The saying "Bad Habits Die Hard" is accurate. Because bad habits have been ingrained in our bodies and minds for a long time, they are challenging to break. On the one hand, we have vices that can endanger our lives, such as smoking and drinking. On the other hand, are some vices that anonymity lifestyles, such as sleeping late, regularly watching late-night television, being attached to social media, etc. c?

Resista? c e to Change: It takes time to break undesirable habits; it cannot be done all at once. It is a gradual procedure that could demand more significant effort than is reasonable. Our bodies may change, and they do so swiftly in the case of poor habits. Our everyday routines turn into habits, and constant repetition strengthens them. Our bodies are not suited to a healthy lifestyle. Thus, there is excellent resistance when we try to change this system. This resistance differs from person to person based on the degree of addiction.

Dependence on Medicines: We don't have time to exercise in our fast-paced society, but we do have time to visit a doctor and receive treatment for our ailments.

Most medications are painkillers; they reduce pain but do not treat the underlying condition or prevent a recurrence. However, we find it more convenient to take medication than to exercise for 30 minutes since we need relief now. Then some individuals are so busy that they cannot seek medical attention and instead turn to over-the-counter medication.

Although medications offer quick respite from our pain and suffering, is this the best action for your health issues? Not. While those with joint problems can eliminate their problems with a simple schedule of regular exercise, those with chronic problems do need personal, professional stive Source of Inspiration.

Although maintaining good health has many advantages, those who criticize healthy lifestyles frequently use them as an alibi for their unhealthy habits. Examples of people who still get ailments while maintaining an exercise schedule. But who knows what stage of an illness one is experiencing, how long it will take to get back to normal, or whether the activity is being done correctly? Then there are those who, despite years of running or walking, still have pot bellies. It should be realized that we make assumptions in this situation since we don't have all the facts.

CHAPTER 7

How can health be made more valuable?

It can be challenging, but it is possible to turn health into wealth. However, performing anything simple to do is fine.

- **Adage:** You must believe in it to strive for it. The most excellent method to make "Health is Wealth" your mantra is to believe it and remind yourself of it frequently. Belief in something makes it possible to achieve it and inspires your efforts. To evoke and inspire a desire to accomplish your goal, listen to, watch, or read health-related media. Think of excellent health as a strategy to achieve success in all spheres of your life. By acting on the initiative, belief is further enhanced.

- **Follow the Advice:** We may build a solid foundation for excellent health by following the advice. Nothing unusual needs to be done on your part. Just organize your regimen and stick to it. You must realize that it is an affair at least five to six days a week, if not every day. Simply getting up early and going for a walk, run, or jog is one of the cheapest ways to pursue good health. One merely needs to spend money on a decent pair of shoes. As for exercising the mind, one can meditate by sitting still, keeping their eyes closed, and doing nothing for a minimum of 15 to 30 minutes. There is also the option of praying. Similarly, consume a balanced diet daily with fruits, vegetables, and other nourishing foods. AdditioOnerk out at home using a personal gym, a treadmill, or other equipment.

- **Firm Commitment:** To maintain a healthy lifestyle, one must make a firm commitment that lasts a lifetime rather than just a week or a month. At first, for a day or a week, we are all fired up. After that, we resume our sedentary way of life if one's health should be taken care of continuously rather than in stages. We must adhere to a regimen of exercise and healthy eating. To firmly resolve, never to give up, and to k, keep trying, no matter how many times you might fail. Motivate yourself by engaging in a regular exercise routine. Please pay attention to the pattern and follow it. If necessary, add your ideas. Another option is to join a friend or acquaintance in a fitness regimen. Doing this will motivate you to stick with it since you are now a team and accountable to one another. Make your flaws, fear of getting sick, or anything else that can be a source of dedication.

- **Please don't push yourself too hard:** Often, we have all we need to stay healthy, but we lack the motivation or don't use the skills correctly. Avoid taking things too seriously or hastily because doing so could have unfavorable effects. You are not competing; take it easy. In a frenzy, we frequently overdo certain things that wear us out or make us sick. The ideal course of action is to start small and build intensity and duration until you reach a suitable platform. Avoid attempting too many things at once; concentrate on one specific exercise. Keep in mind that "Slow and Steady Wins the Race."

- **Change your Lifestyle:** A change in your lifestyle positively impacts your health. Sometimes all it takes to improve our health is a simple shift in habits, like going to bed and waking up early. This regimen by itself gives us plenty of time to balance our activities. Then, we can modify the type and amount of our diet to meet personal needs. It's not required to consume whatever the family consumes. Based on consultation with a nutritionist or doctor, eat what suits you the best. Bring a healthy balance throughout your career, physical health, interpersonal relationships, financial situation, spirituality, surroundings, and all other factors. Only indulge in your sluggish habits once a week to avoid getting bored with your existing schedule.

- **Seek Professional Assistance:** Some people need a push or a set of circumstances to drive themselves to live a healthy lifestyle. Nutritionists, personal trainers, fitness experts, rehabilitative professionals, fitness coaches, gyms, and other professionals can enhance this effort.

Since many of us have not decided where to begin or what to do, professional assistance is valuable and suitable. We are encouraged to follow our professional and regular mind for our health because we know that we have invested money and don't want it wasted.

- **Access Health Resources:** There are many ways to acquire access to health-related information, including books, DVDs, electronic devices, machinery, periodicals, newspapers, television, radio, the internet, and so on. Some are inexpensive and simple to find online, in libraries, and on television, while others are pricey. Aerobics Videos are accessible in video stores, online, and on television for those who cannot exercise outside or find it difficult. These offer fitness plans that are quickly followed by just mimicking the routines. To augment your current health program, read the health articles, follow them, and apply particular technology.

- **Bring Variations:** After a while, some activities lose effectiveness or stop keeping us as healthy as we should or want them to. Find different sources of exercise instead, or change your routine. If you're bored, you can engage in other activities that positively impact your health and offer a new perspective. Try new things and be inventive by combining two or three healthy activities. You can combine exercise with daily tasks like cleaning a room rhythmically to make it more fascinating or playing a game of cricket or chess if that's something you last did a while ago. You can also add variety to your daily routine by occasionally riding a bike to work instead of driving. These modest actions have a significant impact.

- **Be your mentor:** We frequently enroll our friends in fitness programs, and it frequently happens that their interest wanes after a while. Here, peer influence might cause us to lose focus on our objectives, feel alone, or become frustrated when our chosen partner backs out or loses interest. Always remember that you will stick to your schedule in this situation. Be independent, don't rely too heavily on others, and realize that your relationship might not last forever. Instead, enjoy it while it lasts.

Think This out this Basic Self-Care Advice:

In addition to the absence of sickness in the body, good health also refers to a person's physical, mental, social, and spiritual well-being.

Exercising for at least 30 minutes per day, such as walking, jogging, or running.

Five (5) minutes every day, on average, of deep breathing exercises meditation.

Take brief breaks when necessary.

Choose the people you spend time with carefully each day.

Each day, find something to giggle about.

Consume a balanced diet that is high in veggies.

Give up emotional eating.

Start a journal and record at least one happy memory from each day.

Developing the ability to say "No" to others while saying "Yes" to yourself.

Make time to rest.

Weekend self-care getaway.

Go outside and take in the scenery.

Don't wait; take care of your needs for self-care right away!

Starting a self-care habit is always early enough. The global epidemic has even highlighted the importance of health in all its facets. Look for simple methods to immediately incorporate self-care into your daily life so you can keep your health.